THE
BLUFFER'S GUIDE®
TO
DOCTORING

PATRICK KEATING

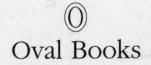

Oval Books

Published by Oval Books
335 Kennington Road
London SE11 4QE
United Kingdom

Telephone: +44 (0)20 7582 7123
Fax: +44 (0)20 7582 1022
E-mail: info@ovalbooks.com

First published by Ravette Publishing, 1993
Reprinted 1994,1997

New edition published by Oval Books, 1999
Updated 2000

Series Editor – Anne Tauté

Cover designer – Jim Wire, Quantum
Printer – Cox & Wyman Ltd
Producer – Oval Projects Ltd

The Bluffer's Guides® series is based
on an original idea by Peter Wolfe.

The Bluffer's Guide®, The Bluffer's
Guides®, Bluffer's®, and Bluff Your
Way® are Registered Trademarks.

ISBN: 1-902825-05-5

CONTENTS

INTRODUCTION

Doctoring, the art of practising medicine, as distinct from neutering the family pet, is a skill that some seem to acquire effortlessly. The less fortunate majority of medical graduates find themselves terminally confused before they have taken their graduation gown back to Moss Bros.

There are definite ground rules and *'modi operandi'* which dawn as the years pass but these are not passed down because part of the fun is watching the 'new blood' run around like lobotomised chickens. This is known as 'character-building' in the trade and the practice dates from Roman times when they used to throw the Christians to the lions.

One of the questions asked *ad nauseam* at interviews for prospective medical students is 'Were either of your parents doctors?' Either this is a straight memory test or it implies that there is some genetic predisposition towards the noble art. More likely the question is aimed at finding out if the aged parents can afford the fees.

Prospective entrants into medical school are usually asked for high grades of passes at 'A' level. This perpetuates the myth that doctors are extremely bright – a rumour most likely to have been started by a doctor in the first place. Medical students would be more accurately described as above average 'grafters' who will be able to assimilate the sheer volume of facts and information required. They are the 'mules' of the university student body and Mensa members are pretty thin on the ground. If they were that bright they would have researched what they were getting into a bit better and gone into the Civil Service.

Another question asked of prospective entrants is 'Why do you want to do Medicine?' At this point candidates' eyes usually roll upwards and moisten as they give the monastic reply, 'I want to help people'. This stirs the memories of the interviewing panel as they recall giving that exact same reply half a century earlier. The nostalgia cycle is complete and the medical novice is sent home to pack his or her bags.

This optimism usually survives the five harrowing years of training and after graduation most fledgling doctors are still eager and straining at the leash to start their future careers.

This slender tome and coffee table 'must' is intended to give the aspiring medico a glance at the opposition, some of the rules and pitfalls and a few of the tactics used by the more experienced. Thus armed, you will tread through your future career as sure of foot as a blindfolded steel erector in high heels.

FAMOUS FOREBEARS

Doctoring in its earliest form probably began in pre-historic times when an unlucky hunter, after getting on the wrong side of some wild beast, would shout in desperation 'Medic!' Then some enterprising and caring soul, later identified as Homo Medicus, would rush to the scene, giving the now familiar rhythmical cry 'Nee-naw, nee-naw' and attend to his injuries on the spot or drag him back for more prolonged treatment in his Intensive Cave Unit.

The most successful early doctors kept their skills shrouded in mystery and performed their rituals with flair and style. While under a full moon, they might give the client a toad to suck three times a day, quickly followed by a bill for half his year's earnings, preferably in a language he couldn't understand. All that remained to do then was for him to sit back and wait for someone to invent the Volvo Estate and a set of golf clubs.

In the Middle Ages there were many disputes as to who was a physician and who wasn't. There were numerous 'allied trades' – leechers, bladder stone cutters, boil lancers and barbers getting in on the act and spoiling it for those who had done their proper apprenticeship in the healing arts. The confused public came off worse as they had no way of knowing whether they were baring their all to the genuine article or someone who did 'doctoring' for beer money.

Much later in Britain, in 1858, the 'Medical Act' declared that all persons acting as bogus doctors would be fined £20. Today, interest in the 'quasi medical disciplines' of homeopathy, acupuncture, chiropracting, osteopathy, reflexology and herbalism is gaining strength again. Holistic medicine, treating the person as a 'whole', has a place but you wouldn't have much use for it in an emergency. When was the last time you heard an urgent request for a feng shui expert over a loudspeaker?

Now that you are properly qualified in the healing arts, it's your turn to don the ceremonial white coat. Whether for reasons of wisdom or a typing error, your medical school has ennobled you with the lofty title of 'Dr'. Strictly speaking, in Britain, this is an honorary title as most medically qualified people possess the degree of 'Bachelor of Medicine' and not an MD. This minor detail will make absolutely no difference to your mother who has been telling all and sundry that you were going to be a doctor ever since you were in short pants.

As a fellow 'medic', you are in rare company indeed. Here are some caring professionals, past and present, who share this medical title with you. As you will see, not all would make good role models.

Hippocrates (460 BC)

The 'Father of Medicine' and a Greek from the island of Kos. He is accredited as the founder of modern medical principles. Amongst other things, he advised his patients to pray and wash and make sacrifices in order to get better, which still holds true today in the National Health Service.

He published the first findings on the serious after-effects of the week-old doner kebab.

He was probably the first doctor to advocate the use of foul language (the Hippocratic Oath), and all doctors are required by law to do the same at all times in moments of frustration.

Dr William Harvey English Physician (1578-1657)

He was the first doctor to realise that blood went round and round. He described the circulation of the blood through arteries and veins and explained the heart's action with the use of valves. In order to show this, he experimented with a lot of very nervous horses, some buckets and probably an exceedingly large shovel.

His research revolutionised medical thinking but it was later discredited after a steward's enquiry.

Dr Edward Jenner English Physician (1749-1823)

The pioneer of vaccination who saved people from smallpox by giving them cowpox. This all came about because he noticed that those working in the vicinity of dairy cattle escaped the worst ravishes of the killer disease.

He worked tirelessly in developing his 'vaccination' with a lot of dairymaids and thus became a real star in the pox department.

Dr Joseph Lister Scottish surgeon (1827-1912)

He introduced the practice of 'antisepsis' by using dressings soaked in carbolic acid to kill off bacteria. Prior to this many people died from infection following surgery. Until this discovery, if patients were told they were having an operation, a priest would be called for at the same time.

Carbolic acid was a kind of primitive and inexpensive 'antibiotic'. Hospital tea is now thought to work on the same principle.

Dr John Snow English Anaesthetist (1813-58)

This early 19th-century doctor was a first-footer on the road to painless medicine and became a pioneer in the field of what is now called 'anaesthetics' which literally means 'without feelings'. Prior to his discoveries, the only way anyone endured the pain of surgery was to get commode-hugging drunk.

He somewhat bravely gave chloroform to Queen Victoria in 1853 for the birth of her eighth child, Prince Leopold. The method gained some popularity as 'chloroform à la reine' and the sovereign was so pleased with the pain-free experience that she requested it for the conception of her ninth so she could lie back and think of nothing.

Dr Marie Stopes Birth Controller (1880-1958)

One of the first women doctors. A true feminist and asserter of the woman's right to plan her family. She wrote the *Guide to Married Love* in 1918, which must have been a real welcome home for the love-starved troops from the trenches in France.

Dr Benjamin Spock Paediatrician (1903-98)

This now famous American wrote his *Common Sense Book of Baby and Child Care* in 1946 which advocated less rigidity in bringing up children. Mothers at the time went completely overboard and permissiveness became the rule so that an entire generation wandered around in the 1960s covered in body paint and smoking pot.

Dr Richard Gordon Author (1921)

In real life an anaesthetist at St Bartholomew's Hospital, London, and one-time ship's surgeon, he wrote 34 novels and non-fiction books, plus the famous *Doctor in the House* series which launched Dirk Bogarde to fame in the eponymous films and glamourised doctoring for a generation of youngsters.

Dr Alex Comfort Sexologist

He gave the doctor's stamp of approval to imaginative procreation in his worthy and trendy tome *The Joy of Sex*. This showed some positions for athletic coition that would make a contortionist cry. He is now rumoured to be writing the much needed sequel for practitioners, 'The Joy of Traction'.

Other famous doctors include Dr Christiaan Barnard, Sir Arthur Conan Doyle, Dr Roger Bannister the four minute miler, Dr Anton Chekhov, the playwright, and Drs Zhivago, Kildare, Crippen, Frankenstein, Finlay, Jekyll, Who, McCoy, and No.

QUALIFYING AND BEYOND

A period of numbness affects new doctors that lasts for some time after graduation. This is mainly due to two factors:

1. They actually qualified.
2. They have to start earning a living.

For several weeks afterwards many medical graduates live in dread of learning that the results were mixed up and they have to do their final year over again. It is not the humiliation that bothers them so much as the three months backpacking around the beer halls of Europe that they will be forced to miss.

The average cost of educating a medical student is about £150,000 excluding bar bills, so it is not surprising that they are now expected to do some work for that investment.

If doctors ever want to work abroad there are some extra qualifications that are best taken immediately after the final exams while the memory is still fresh. For some this is just asking too much and they disappear immediately, confident in the fact that their piece of paper bearing witness to their qualifications will, like an American Express Card, be acceptable all over the medical world.

The smart ones who resist this temptation at least take the extra exams to enable them to work, for example in the USA (ECFMG and VQE), speedily present their TTFN (Ta Ta For Now) certificate to the appropriate authority and disappear to do research into suntan injuries on a Californian beach.

For the not-so-smart who missed the chance of being evacuated to sunnier and more lucrative climes, there are years to come of 'blood, sweat and tears', and only some of these will come from the patients.

The Road Ahead (Quo Vadis?)

The basic plan of all the great and not so great medical careers starts in the same way and follows the same early path. It all begins with the ubiquitous and newly qualified **House Officer**, so called because this doctor is so overburdened with work that he never gets to leave the building. This fledgling will struggle for six months in general surgery and six months in general medicine, making a total of twelve months in purgatory.

At the end of each of these 'pre-registration' jobs their consultants will be required to give a reference as to how they fared during this period. Some references are good but most are mediocre and the consultants try and limit themselves to the statement that in their opinion the doctor is unlikely to make any serious gaffs in the near future.

Consultants are not fools: a more confident prediction in writing might result in a lawsuit at a later date. Some references can be so bad as to condemn the house officer to repeat the entire first year again. Occasionally, a reference will have to be read twice to appreciate its full implications, such as: 'Dr Smith tells me that he has worked for me for six months. In that time he has performed his duties entirely to his own satisfaction. I'm sure we would all benefit from seeing him run through them once more.'

Those who survive this bewildering year with satisfactory references are graced with full registration with the doctor's governing body, the **General Medical Council** (GMC).

The period of probation is now officially at an end and most doctors will choose to move further afield, severing their umbilical attachment to anything that even resembles training. The stabilisers are well and truly off the bicycles and they make their way towards a longed-for speciality or head for experience in far flung parts of the world.

Fully registered junior doctors are given the lofty title in their next job of **Senior House Officer** (SHO). At this point they must make a choice as to which speciality would most benefit from their talents. This decision is based almost entirely on their limited exposure to such specialities while a student and a house officer. Judgement here is not entirely rational and may be based on such flimsy observations as 'the consultant in orthopaedic surgery speaks nicely, has a healthy tan, a house in the country and drives a Bentley'. Enter one embryonic orthopaedic surgeon.

Specialising in Something

Broadly speaking, the specialities may be divided into hospital-based practice, General Practice in the community or practice linked to something else such as the pharmaceutical industry or the armed forces or the Department of Health.

There does exist a species of doctor who excels in the theory of medicine but doesn't like the practical stuff where patients are involved. They will often find themselves working permanently in the research field if they are bright enough, or sitting behind a desk in some administrative capacity writing out memos and telling everybody else what to do, if they're not. Nobody knows how many bureaucratic doctors there are behind the scenes until there is something like a national outbreak of Anthrax and they all come out of the woodwork with the appropriate paperwork.

A big shake up in the training of doctors within the specialities has brought the British system into line with European regulations. The most junior specialist is termed **Senior House Officer I** (in case you lose heart). The next position is **Senior House Officer II** from which you progress to the upper level of training and the term **Specialist Registrar**. The reward at the end of the learning curve is **Certificate of Completion of Specialist Training** (CCST), which allows you to become eligible for deification as a Consultant.

This metamorphosis from the newly qualified to the consultant doctor can take place fairly quickly for those adept at taking their specialist exams. Junior doctors tend to fall into two broad groups: those who excel academically and those who excel at day to day 'doctoring' who can't take exams for toffee. There are very few who are good at both. Most doctors take their postgraduate exams at least twice, and sometimes several times, before they either pass or give up and join the Foreign Legion.

The corresponding junior position within General Practice is the **Trainee** who will also have completed at least three years' general training. As the practice junior, they will be expected to work in an office the size of a broom cupboard next to the practice lavatories, and see all the unpopular patients who have been handed down for years.

After they have gained their Membership of the Royal College of General Practitioners, they may rise to the status of **Full Partner** when they will be given a larger room, somewhere to park their car, the pick of the patients and a desk the same size as the room that the new trainee starts in.

CHOOSING A SPECIALITY

To make a choice of career that is going to last for the rest of your working life is daunting. Dermatology or venereology? That is the question.

The amount of advice and guidance available to you in making this important choice could be written on the back of an aspirin and it makes sense here to have a go at a few specialities to see if you like them. However, 'dithering' is frowned upon and the consummate professional will describe these few trial runs as 'broadening the base of their skills' rather than the more truthful 'suck it and see'. Admitting to your boss at the time that, like the Saturday shopper, you are 'just browsing' will be seen at best as less than committed and at worst frivolous.

Such a 'career walkabout' is expected and even encouraged in the Antipodes. Many Australian trainee surgeons get little actual operating experience in their native country and are often sent to 'Practise on the Poms' before they are let loose on their own population.

Going for a professional wander in Britain is considered, though never stated, as unprofessional and 'just not done'. So when, like Dorothy in the *Wizard of Oz*, you suddenly wake up to find yourself committed to Gastroenterology for six months and some solemn old fossil stares down over his bifocals and skewers you with the question 'So you want to specialise in diseases of the bowels do you, doctor?', the answer is "Yes please, sir". Be diplomatic. After all, the poor chap has probably devoted the best years of his life to the art.

For the still undecided, here is a back-of-the-beer-mat guide to what some of the higher profile specialities involve and expect of their devotees.

General Medicine: 'The Physicians' or 'Medics'

Most general physicians will tackle and give expert opinion on just about anything. They are what the purists refer to as the 'proper doctors'. This means that they do most of their work from the bottom of the patient's bed, rarely take their hands out of their pockets and never get them dirty. It is usual for the hospital-based physician to have a special area of interest such as diseases of the heart (Cardiology), the intestines (Gastroenterology) or maybe the diseases of the joints (Rheumatology).

The postgraduate examination to get under your belt as early as possible is the MRCP (Membership of the Royal College of Physicians). It is one of the more difficult exams to pass. If you are thinking of this as the direction for you, then be warned. Applicants are expected to have a brain the size of a basketball and a special interest in obscure and preferably incurable maladies.

If you are something of an infant savant, have discovered bow ties, Clark's shoes with the animal prints on the soles and like train spotting on your weekends off, then this is the one for you.

General Surgery: 'The Cutting Crew'

As their job description states, these surgeons should be able to tackle anything they can get their knife into. In practice they may spend most of their time in a specialist area of surgery such as that of the Urinary System (a Genito-urinary Surgeon), or of the vessels of the body (an Arterial Surgeon).

The exam to sacrifice yourself in the name of here is the dreaded FRCS (Fellow of the Royal College of

Surgeons). Don't be shamed into falling on your
scalpel if you don't pass first time. This is another
hard one where you can be failed for having your tie
on crooked.

When doctors become members of this college,
tradition requires that they lose the title of 'Dr' and
become a 'Mr' again. God knows why, after all the
trouble they went to in the first place. So if a
colleague comes back from taking exams at the Royal
College declaring that he is a 'Mr' now, buy him a
drink. He has either passed or has been disbarred
completely and will need one either way.

Surgeons of the future should bear in mind that
any sized brain is permitted at a push, but you will be
expected to have the same attacking instinct as the
Real Madrid forward line.

In addition, you should profess a disturbing if not
morbid interest in finding out how things work by
taking them apart, and merely a passing interest in
putting them back together again.

Orthopaedic Surgery: 'The Orthopods'

Having grown from the early days of 'straightening
children' (lit. Orthopaedic), this area of surgery is
confined to the skeleton of the body. Its practitioners
spend most of their time resetting fractured bones
and redesigning people's hips and knees and dealing
with the results of trauma.

The instruments that are used in this speciality are
more like earth-moving apparatus compared with the
precision tools used in other areas of surgery. These
surgeons are expected to have the 'Fellowship' exam
but get an additional medal emblazoned with a saw
and crossed bones.

As a general guide for suitability, if you can't read this sentence without moving your lips then this could be the subject for you. Here you will be expected to be as strong as an ox and about twice as intelligent. Showing that you remember any of your medical training apart from how the skeleton fits together will be viewed with grave suspicion.

Take time to re-learn your Meccano skills and be prepared to mould more plaster of Paris than Rodin ever saw in his entire life. Honours marks are usually awarded weekly for anyone guiding the orthopaedic team to the appropriate bed, and marking the patient's limbs with 'R' and 'L', as appropriate, will be seen as having a definite flair for the subject.

Cardiac/Brain Surgery: 'Heart and Soul'

These highly specialised surgeons boldly go where no other surgeons in their right mind would dare. Both types of surgery have only become commonplace with the advent of specialised pumping machinery that enables the work of the heart to be by-passed.

Heart surgeons can now transplant just about anything into anyone. When the brain surgeons manage to do the same thing, what will they do with the donors?

Being one of these specialists is not a career for the half-hearted, and culturing your ego to the size of Big Ben will be an enormous advantage. The surgical skills required are not extraordinary, but the powers of endurance are. Some operations last an exhausting 12 hours or more and while you are busy saving the patient's capacity to circulate blood and reason with the world, you will be rapidly losing yours.

Cosmetic Surgery: 'The Facemakers'

Forget heart transplants, appendicectomies, hip replacements and other routine life-saving surgical procedures performed by lesser beings: as far as you're concerned, surgery is skin deep.

As a master of the 'fantastic plastic' you will possess the uncanny ability to look at someone with a face like the back end of a rhinoceros (aesthetically challenged) and see the potential beauty beneath, only awaiting your skills and hours of painful surgery, followed by six months looking like the Invisible Man and sucking lunch through a straw.

A flair with 'before' and 'after' photos is vital. Most successful cosmetic surgeons with an eye to the 'showbiz' market will have a signed photograph of someone like Barbara Cartland in their office to show that being dead for over ten years is no barrier to looking good.

Radiology: 'The X-ray Doctors'

All doctors who qualified after X-rays were discovered (by Röntgen in 1895) should be able to glean a modest amount of information from these dreary black and white pictures that almost all patients have taken when they arrive in hospital. Modern computerised technology has brought the CAT and MRI scanners where the poor patient disappears into a giant washing machine for about 40 minutes (longer if you add a conditioned rinse). Radiologists are experts, however, at taking and interpreting these films. Show them the picture of a man's skull and they will tell you when he last had a shave.

If you are prepared to risk getting 'rickets' from the

lack of sunlight, and like sitting in dark rooms all day looking at X-Ray (not X-rated) films, then this speciality might prove attractive. In application, previous experience behind the holiday snaps counter at *Boots* will be worth a mention.

Promotion, if not stardom, will be assured if you can come up with any diagnosis from a picture that looks to the uninitiated like an airborne photo of the East London docks taken at night.

Neurology: 'The Nervous Doctors'

This erudite area of general medicine deals with diseases of the brain and nervous system of the body. In order to elicit the signs of these diseases the accomplished neurologist carries around various instruments and tools of torture. Rummage through their pockets and you will find pins for sticking in patients and little toffee hammers for tapping their kneecaps.

As a budding member of this speciality you may be called upon to sort out some pretty weird spasms, tics and all manner of bizarre syndromes. When faced with something that has you completely foxed, the knack is to give the whole thing an impressive German-sounding name, prescribe the human equivalent of Bob Martin's, thank everybody concerned for such an interesting case and then go to lunch.

Obstetrics and Gynaecology: 'Obs and Gobs'

This area is the medicine of the female reproductive system including the end product, namely the birth of babies. It is really a specialised area of general medicine and surgery.

Increasingly, and some would say quite rightly, this is becoming a service 'for women by women' surgeons. However things change very slowly in medicine and there are still many men devoted to this subject.

Membership of the Royal College of Obstetricians and Gynaecologists is your aim and it is said that the sort of doctor who succeeds in this speciality has the ability to wallpaper their hall through their letterbox.

As a career choice, only masochists and those who thrive on sleep deprivation should consider this one. Emerging babies have no regard for the phenomenon of the normal working day and prefer to arrive in the middle of the night. At the end of six months of this you'll look like one of the Addams family. Volunteering for longer than this is tantamount to insanity.

Anaesthetics: 'The Gas Men'

This is a relatively new area of medical expertise which has only been recognised as a speciality for about 50 years. Before that time, anybody who happened to be passing by might be asked to pour ether or chloroform over a handkerchief to keep the patient comatose. Before that, there was nothing to pour on the hanky.

Today all anaesthetists, over and above their general medical training, become experts in applied pharmacology (how drugs work) and applied physiology (how the body's systems work). However, if you want to render a Gas Man speechless, ask "How much longer would you have to train to become a proper doctor?"

As a trainee anaesthetist you enter a much maligned area of medical accomplishment whose artisans, like medical sandmen, drug their trusting

subjects through somewhat arduous surgical procedures. They possess a wry, if somewhat macabre,
sense of humour and are renowned experts at the
Daily Telegraph crossword, probably because some of
their patients are still awake enough to help them
with the tricky bits.

A spell in the hi-tech environment of the Intensive
Care Unit will be required at some time in your training, so prepare for this experience by going there in
your spare time, dismantling some wizard piece of
life-saving apparatus and then saying nonchalantly,
"Sister, could you fix this please?", and swiftly leaving
the room.

Paediatrics: 'The Baby Doctors'

The medicine of children and especially babies is not
simply 'scaled down' adult medicine. It is a totally
different game.

When an adult becomes ill, the doctor usually has a
little time to stand around and scratch his head and
think, but with children things can deteriorate much
more rapidly and one can become seriously unglued.
It's almost like dealing with a different species, and
you might as well throw away the anatomical and
physiological rule book that took so long to learn.

This is a very competitive area of medicine and you
will need the Membership of The Royal College of
Physicians and the Diploma in Child Health (DCH)
under your belt if you wish to make it your career.
Something happens to doctors when they are sur-
rounded by children all the time, so be prepared to
mutate from the skilled professional image to the
shambling, avuncular or eccentric auntie type.

Empathy with your junior patients is the flavour of

the moment. The modern approach is to forget the white coat and to cover yourself in teddy bear badges to gain the toddlers' confidence prior to making cooing noises and sticking needles in them.

The one in the nylon shirt, clashing kipper tie and crimplene flares, with the gonk pen on a thong around his neck, is your consultant.

Venereology: 'The Pox Doctors'

Venereologists are, in the main, general physicians who, for reasons best known to themselves, specialise in the troublesome trouser ailments of the adult reproductive and plumbing systems. It all comes under the title of 'GUM', an unfortunate and tasteless abbreviation, which stands for genito-urinary medicine.

The layman will refer to this shady emporium of expertise as the 'Clap Clinic' in the saloon and the 'Special Clinic' in the lounge. Either way, it is spoken of in hushed tones and nobody likes to have to go there. Appropriately, just like some speakeasy selling bootleg penicillin, this department is usually located discreetly at the back of the hospital.

If you are a pillar of the church, have led a sheltered life thus far and think that 'intercourse' means the same thing as 'conversation', then this may not be the area for you.

Pathology: 'The Dead Right Doctors'

Pathologists study the process and progression of diseases. They can tell you just about everything that happens in a disease but only when it's too late and the patient is no more.

They are in the enviable position, medically speaking, of being able to have a good ferret round at their leisure, knowing that the patient is not going to get any worse. This is the domain of the 20-20 hindsight merchants. At post mortems they must not only tell their colleagues where they went wrong in their diagnoses but do it with glee, in a loud voice, and relish their listeners' embarrassment. A fondness for asking impossible questions to those ignorant medical students who are still conscious is mandatory.

You will of course be expected to become a fully embalmed member of the Royal College of Pathologists. No squeamishness is permitted, and any aspiring pathologist should be able to decant gastric contents into a bucket of giblets while eating a chicken tikka sandwich and thinking of the summer holidays with the kids at the same time.

Psychiatry: 'The Trick Cyclists' or 'Freud Squad'

Most psychiatrists worth their salt will acknowledge that they are a strange bunch. If you are curious about the workings of the mind and not too bothered about the state of your own, a spell here will do you no harm. But if you are one of those who feel that people claiming to hear strange voices in their heads should give themselves a good talking to, then think again.

Even the most consummate of medical bluffers should be wary of entering this realm of soft couches and glazed eyes lest they end up in a rubber room themselves. As a general rule, the best thing to do if you get an idea like becoming a psychiatrist is to swallow your own weight in tranquillisers and lie down till it goes away.

There are many more hospital specialities to try, and moving around all the 'ologies' could be a career in itself. However, while this might make your CV look as impressive as the Dead Sea Scrolls, you would run the risk of being branded as something of a medical itinerant.

MEDICAL HIERARCHY

Medical personnel in a hospital have a well recognised rank system and, as in the armed forces, everybody is supposed to know their place.

Their uniforms are not obvious but their style is. Remember that even as a relatively inexperienced doctor you have an important place in what is now trendily referred to as the 'Health Care Team'. You are a cog in a well oiled machine. But take care, some cogs are definitely oilier than others.

As the ladder of seniority is scaled, so the memory of what it was like to be a 'junior doctor' fades. In some senior medical icons, the memory of what it was like to be a mere human being fades altogether.

The term 'junior' here is usually applied to any doctor up to the grade of Specialist Registrar. If you have any difficulty in thinking where you fit in, then the following classification may be of some help.

Professor

Only in teaching hospitals do you have professors. They are consultant grade doctors who are responsible for an entire department devoted to a speciality. Thus you will have a Professor of Surgery, Medicine, Psychiatry and so forth. The largest establishments can have professors in all sorts of obscure subjects. Usually the bigger the title, the smaller the speciality and, more importantly, the teaching of that speciality to doctors in training and medical students.

A professor may sometimes hold a 'Chair' in a particular subject. The holding of a chair is not only a testament to upper body strength, it is a bestowed honour and often carries an important name and a small stipend to go with it. This can give their title added flair and clout, such as the 'King Herod Professor of Paediatrics' or, one that whiffs of commercial sponsorship, the 'ICI Professor of Plastic Surgery'.

In Britain it used to be customary to be a museum piece before you reached this rank and was seen as a chivalrous method of promoting consultants up and out of the way. Like Captain Oates, they could say 'I'm just popping off to be a professor. I may be some time'; and quietly disappear behind a pile of books, never to be seen again. However, there is now emerging a new superbreed of trainee specialist. Those who seem to have a flair for original thinking, conducting research and teaching their subject are encouraged to become **lecturers** within the university. Custom then dictates that they go round and round, researching and teaching and then scrabbling with the competition for the chair of their choice when the music stops.

Consultant

Consultants are universally recognised by staff and patients alike to be 'a little higher than the angels'. Once this title has been bestowed, the power they wield is awesome. They are doctors who have risen through the ranks to the top of their speciality. These 'Superdocs', like Superman, can leap insurmountable medical catastrophes at a single bound and are faster than a locomotive, especially if they have to go and play golf or get the Daimler serviced. Patients always know who the consultants are by the fact that they dress smartly, have clean fingernails, don't look tired all the time and aren't loaded down with notes.

When taken to the bedside and tactfully 'reminded' of the salient facts about a patient, they have the disturbing knack of asking their staff just the right (read wrong) questions for which they don't have answers. They are rumoured to talk directly with God about matters that need not concern the rest of us. Ask any patients who their consultant is and they will usually beam and add proudly to the name that he is 'the top man in his field'. As a small reward for being ultimately responsible for the welfare of the patients they have their names emblazoned over the victim's bed.

Modes of behaviour for consultants vary from the benevolent to the tyrannical. Junior staff would be wise to get to read these moods quickly. If in doubt, stick close to the ward sister. If you're really lucky she will be an experienced one who has been around for a while and who remembers your consultant when he was a medical student.

All have their hobby horses that must be perfectly adhered to by their junior staff. Once these foibles have been spotted and mastered, your life will be easier. However, it's a bit like painting the Forth Bridge: once you've got them worked out, it's time to move on and start all over again. When consultants go to heaven, God must have a really hard job convincing them that it's time to take a back seat.

Specialist Registrar

These are specialists in training who have passed the required exams and have about another three years to go before gaining the certification necessary to be Consultants. They may know their subject but have a lot to bone up on about management issues, committees and all the vital street-fighting skills necessary to survive in the real world of hospital practice.

Generally they have not forgotten what it was like to be a doctor in training and can quite often be disarmingly human. But when the consultant is away from the hospital at some World Conference on Scrofula in Hawaii, they may deputise for, or more accurately play at being, Attila the Hun.

Senior House Officer II

Once called Registrars, these doctors are middle ranking trainee specialists who are the workhorses of the hospital wards. They are always either working for an exam or recovering from a recent bruising encounter with the examiners.

Add to this the mental exhaustion of being constantly on call, about half a kilo of bleeps to carry and a library of patients' notes, and the bleary-eyed result is the keen, on-the-ball professional that every patient would want on their case.

Senior House Officer I

These doctors are junior trainees within a speciality. If you want to know the *theory* of how some medical problem should be dealt with, this is the doctor to ask. If they don't know, they will know which book gives the answer. They are usually boundlessly enthusiastic about their subjects and have to be constantly restrained from doing things that they have only read about in books.

House Officer

These are doctors within their first year of qualifying. They are qualified but unregistered, and they occupy a sort of no man's land in the medical world.

House Wallahs, as they are affectionately known, swing constantly between triumph and despair depending on the day's events. They will be expected to be responsible and show initiative, but must 'instinctively' know when they should ask for advice and assistance. At the beginning of the job, if they are in any doubt as to what is an unacceptable hour to call on consultant advice, a phone call at about 4 a.m. on a Sunday morning to his home usually sorts the matter out.

As relatively inexperienced doctors, it is time that is the main enemy of house officers. There are not enough hours in the day to get all their tasks done and they may often be seen stalking around the wards in the middle of the night doing things that were forgotten earlier. It is not unheard of for patients to be woken in the middle of the night by the house officer to ask them 'Would you like anything to help you to sleep?'

If house officers are called to the ward during the night, look at the way they are dressed. They usually resemble somebody who has grabbed anything wearable to come out of a burning building. A few will arrive looking immaculate no matter what the hour. Top marks for presentation but you wouldn't want them in a hurry. For day wear, the required attire is a stiff new white coat, a stethoscope worn proudly but nonchalantly around the neck and pockets stuffed with enough paraphernalia and reference books to supply a third world medical mission. They invariably bring up the rear of the medical staff ward round, laboriously pushing a trolley full of notes, looking like some ice-cream vendor and are usually, for the time being anyway, about as well informed.

Medical Students

These apprentices are let loose on the hospital wards in their senior years to learn the practical applications of what they learned in the 'pre-clinical' years. As a hard-pressed junior doctor it is a good idea to try to get these gullible souls to perform as many of the menial tasks as possible with the promise that you will put a word in with the examiners for them. You will never meet their examiners but they don't know this so use their paranoia to your advantage.

Patients can't fail to miss them as they walk sheepishly around the wards usually in groups of not less than six for mutual support. If a patient has anything about their case that is even remotely interesting they would be well advised to keep it to themselves. If the word gets out of something like a 'classic heart murmur' there will be queues of students at their bedside with stethoscopes at the ready.

They are easily recognised by their still trendy haircuts and short off-white coats that look as if they have been in a boil wash for a week. The student diet consists mainly of beer and hospital toast which gives them a pale consumptive look which is designed to make the examiners feel sorry for them.

Students are always laden down with books with titles that start with 'Lecture Notes in ...' or large unsavoury albums such as 'A Pictorial Atlas of the Lower Intestine' which they usually save to read next to some unsuspecting little old lady on the bus.

General Practice

Gone are the days when many doctors gravitated into being General Practitioners (GPs) because their hospital training had finished and they could not think of anything better to do. The College of General Practitioners has seen to it that you have to declare an interest early, at birth if possible.

Nowadays, getting places on the hospital training 'schemes' is fiercely competitive. Some doctors, it seems, can't wait to throw their white coats into the laundry basket for the last time and get a little black bag, a pair of brogues and a breath of freedom. Be wary of this rose-tinted image.

Most GP work is very demanding, often more so than hospital based medicine. Practices range from the single-handed country doctor to the large community health centres in most of the big cities with anything up to 3,000 patients per doctor.

Whatever the type of practice, at the earliest opportunity it is important to obtain the type of receptionist who will not let you be 'bothered' by just any old patients, especially sick ones. Someone complaining that they merely 'feel a bit off colour' won't get through the door, and anybody caught using that tired old chestnut 'at death's door' will get at best an 'urgent cancellation' for about two weeks' time. To convince her a home visit is needed by the doctor, the patient will need to be in possession of a signed chitty from the Holy Ghost. These home visits are done by GPs after the end of surgery for that day and are known as 'Rounds'. Stamina is needed here, at the end of a busy day, to climb broken gates, sprint past angry dogs and fend off hordes of snotty-nosed kids who want to see what you've got in your bag.

Paradoxically, it is this variety and sense of challenge that makes a GP's life worth while. They may be treating a case of measles in a child in one house and then have to gallop next door to attend the home delivery of a baby on the 15th floor of a block of flats with no lift. Such community doctors think that the hospital specialists have an easy time of it with their support staff, their hi-tech back-up services and all their patients conveniently under one roof.

Hospital doctors, on the other hand, would give their patient's right arm to lead the GP's life of cavorting round the countryside and chatting with old ladies over a cup of tea. That is, of course, when they aren't shooting pheasants or playing golf.

Research

At least one piece of research, preferably bearing fruit, is expected to be done by a doctor in training for a hospital speciality.

Research is difficult to do (*ergo* character-building) and therefore essential. It should be new, original and reach the parts of medical knowledge that others have failed to reach. The ideal piece of research should be of Nobel Prize winning standard, change the face of modern medicine as we know it and cost about ten quid. In these times of stringent economy within the health service, this is a difficult task. Gone are the days when some charity-based organisation would stump up loads of money for some doctor who fancies a year off to dispatch more rats than were lost in the Black Death only to come up with some new idea for a verruca cream at the end of it.

A way round this is to try and touch the large pharmaceutical companies for funding. Be warned however, they will probably expect you to wear their company logo on the back of your white coat for a whole year. The results of your research are then published as a 'paper' in some medical journal and bingo, you are an authority on the subject.

Some specialists become mesmerised by seeing their work in print and have hundreds of papers bearing their name. About two or three would do when applying for a consultancy post. More than this might embarrass those on the appointment committee who may only have one good paper and an anonymous letter to the *Sunday Express* between them.

Private Practice

This is mostly the province of consultants but this need not stop you dreaming. A bit of after hours touting and you too can have a private office that looks like a breakfast TV studio.

It is done in all the specialities, especially for what may be termed the 'personal maladies' such as haemorrhoids or for cosmetic surgery where discretion is assured. Most of this 'PP' work takes place in private hospitals with carpets in the foyer so thick that you could lose a shoe in them. They usually have exclusive sounding names like 'The Guinevere Clinic'.

The procedure most commonly performed in all private practice is the partial or total walletectomy.

JOB HUNTING

Junior doctors' job contracts last at the most four years, and some are for only six months at a time so job hunting is 'open season' and a popular pastime. When you have just mastered what is expected of you in one appointment it will be time to search, apply and interview for the next job of your career.

This feeling of being 'permanently temporary' is naturally considered to be very character-building. All job vacancies in Britain are advertised in the *British Medical Journal*, either in the classified section or, in the case of more senior appointments, the *Obituary* columns. If you fancy a speciality, it's best to get yourself attached to a **Training Scheme**, where your training will be organised for you.

If you aren't part of a scheme, ideally your next job should be arranged to follow smoothly on when your present one comes to an end. This doesn't always run to plan and, at some time in their careers, most doctors find themselves taking an unexpected (and unpaid) holiday by being a **Locum**. This is a temporary position which covers doctors who may be sick or on maternity leave or on holiday. It is not recommended to make a career out of doing these locums but try and adopt a positive approach to this gypsy existence.

Life as a wandering understudy can be fun and you can find yourself standing in for a GP on holiday for a week in Widnes or working in a big city heart surgery unit the next. The rate of pay is slightly higher than normal and the responsibility is minimal. So if you accidentally amputate the wrong couple of toes one week, by the time they have got the bandages off to discover the mistake you will have gone before they can say 'Who was that masked man?'

Compiling a CV

On paper you are where you've worked. There is a vast amount of snobbery and name-dropping attached to where you trained, though rivalry is less rampant since the arranged marriage of several of the great London medical schools including such time-honoured bastions of teaching as Guy's Hospital with St Thomas' – the prima donna behaviour of the latter's graduates giving rise to the nickname 'Guys and Dolls'. However, being a mediocre doctor in a prestige establishment in a capital city still carries more weight than being a superb doctor in St Sympathy in the sticks.

That is the system and it is unlikely to change. If you haven't managed to get to Eton and the Guards, acquired honours from Oxford or Cambridge, passed all your exams first time and got the Croix de Guerre in your holidays, don't despair. The contents of your CV and your application form are what gets you on to a shortlist to be interviewed for a job.

Rumour has it that selecting people for a job shortlist is very tedious as is the interviewing process itself. Most people have very similar qualifications or they would not be applying in the first place. Thus your CV should contain something which makes you stand out from the crowd and emphasise your individuality. If you were a catcher in a trapeze act before you went to medical school, flaunt it. They will probably interview you just to see if you have arms like an orang-utan.

Interviews

Once shortlisted, the worst thing you can do is to research the other candidates. You are bound to find that one of them has a PhD from Harvard, has published more papers than Rupert Murdoch and is rumoured to be up for a knighthood. This will not help you to shine on the day.

As for apparel, wear something uncontroversial and avoid college ties. Moustaches and beards are very suspect, especially on women. If you are desperate enough you might try telling all the other nervous hopefuls that the interviews are being held in another building then walk in and say that you're the only one who has turned up.

It is easier to advise what not to say to the usual questions. The teaser asked every time is 'What makes you want to apply for this particular job?' Experienced interview veterans will always avoid the honest and instant riposte: 'A large overdraft, rising damp and two kids to support.'

Exams

Whoever devised the postgraduate exam system for doctors had no respect whatsoever for the Geneva Convention. The technical term used to describe them by most aspiring candidates is 'a real bugger'.

The amount to be learned is vast and must be done at the end of your working day or in the holidays. As the ugly date looms this gives rise to doctors looking like perished elastic bands, unable even to remember who invented the surgical support.

An instant diagnosis of PMS (Pre Matriculation Syndrome) should be made and the patient sedated and put to bed for about two months.

In the examination hall you will be expected to write about five biros' worth of essays, answer hundreds of multiple choice questions and then while your hand (and brain) are still numb you will be marched in front of some patient who has been commissioned for you to examine.

If you are especially unfortunate you will get one who behaves as if trained by the SAS to resist interrogation. Having asked politely as to the nature of their ailment you will get the stone-faced reply, 'You tell me, you're the doctor' or, worse still, 'They told me not to give you any clues.' The examiners, who go around in pairs for safety reasons, can then take great delight in finding out exactly what you don't know.

If your tormentors have had a fortified lunch, unsuccessful candidates may even have the bad news broken to them with what passes for wit. While pointing out of the window they might hear 'Do you see those green leaves on that tree, doctor? Why don't you come back and see us again when they're brown?'

Those destined to repeat the performance leave via a discreet side entrance near a sign that says 'Book Early To Avoid Disappointment'.

The heroic few who have passed the ordeal are invited to meet the examiners and get a drop of cooking sherry. After that lot, you would think they would give you the Victoria Cross.

WHO'S WHO IN HOSPITALS

Apart from the medical staff, there is a whole army of people needed to run a modern hospital. Let's start with the most important.

Car Park Attendant

With this man on the job, you don't stand a chance of parking within the same postal district as the main entrance unless you happen to be a beer lorry delivering to the social club or, at a push, an ambulance.

These monitors of the front gate are invariably victims of a personality disorder. They have a chestful of medals won for having cars towed away beyond the call of duty, and all answers to your pleading start with 'It's more than my job's worth'.

Catering Manager (or Chef de Canteen)

These hospital gourmets are responsible for feeding patients and staff alike. They used to be known as 'the face that launched a thousand chips'. Gone are the hospital curries that could clean out somebody's bowels better than any antibiotic. Nowadays, after a short spell in the Lucrezia Borgia Catering College, they can provide space-age junk food in small enough portions to render the patient's bowels completely redundant until they get home.

The same low residue principle works for the staff too. If you don't have to answer the call of nature so often, you can answer your bleep more.

This is the era of 'caring cuisine': all disabilities are catered for so everything is colour-coded (meat grey, vegetables khaki) for the hard of tasting. Low fat gurus will be impressed by the steamed toast.

Porters

These amiable shire horses of the hospital will shift anything anywhere, providing you have the right chit for it. They will often give the patients the impromptu benefit of their experience while pushing their trolley or wheelchair through the corridors. Try as you might to convince the patient otherwise, they will remember the porter's trenchant comment on the way to X-Ray, 'I pushed a guy once who had that done. He never recovered.'

Switchboard

The operators here used to have a reputation for being abrupt and uncaring. They would leave you hanging in mid-air on the phone with no explanation, or put you through to the chiropodist when you clearly asked for the artificial limb department.

Things are better now because you can listen to twenty minutes of Handel's water music played on a child's stylophone while they put you through to the wrong department.

When you are on duty they are your vital link with any social calls from the outside world, so it pays to be nice to them. At Christmas they usually expect an expensive bottle of something festive from the medical staff in return for their benevolence. Most doctors would agree that to complement their communicating skills a better gift would be hearing aids all round and free speech therapy vouchers.

Hospital Radio

This form of radiotherapy is broadcast incessantly throughout the hospital usually from some boxroom next to the surgical appliances department by some character with a lisp or loose dentures and a fondness for Jim Reeves records.

Get your birthday mentioned here between 'Mrs Smith's varicose veins healing nicely in Crippen Ward' and the third rendering of 'Distant Drums' for the Ear, Nose and Throat department, and your fame will be ensured.

Ward Sister

The most senior nurse in a department or a ward can range from the benign and helpful to the type who thinks that doctors just get in the way.

Any wise new-born doctors will resist the temptation to give the impression that they have been on the job for years. A full confession to the fact that you bring a completely uncluttered mind to the actual practice of medicine will get you a long way.

The benevolent kind of ward sister can assist you in your job, kindly point out any cock-ups and teach you all the things they forgot to tell you in medical school. Conversely, the nightmarish Oberwardführer breed of sister terrifies staff and patients alike and probably only went into nursing because she was considered too antisocial for the Baader-Meinhof gang.

These are usually the ones you meet at two o'clock in the morning when creeping out of the nurses home. What is called for here is not bluffing, but a deft turn of speed.

Hospital Hairdressers (and Beauty Therapists)

These are what remained when the doctors left the Barber-Surgeons union. Their maxim would seem to be that being at death's door in a hospital bed is no obstacle to looking well groomed.

For the ladies a new hairdo, usually bright pink or blue, a full facial and a good douse of *Evening in Paris* is mandatory prior to a consultant ward round. The men can have any style they want as long as it was popular with the enlisted troops in 1940.

Part of their duties used to be to shave patients of any inconvenient body hair prior to having surgery. This practice has been stopped now, probably because patients were taking too long to decide if they would be needing anything for the weekend.

Hospital hairdressers are at their busiest on the day prior to surgery as patients have their new perm done then, so as to look their best on the operating table.

Hospital Managers

These are the modern-day equivalent of the now defunct Matron, with the same sweeping powers, but the well-groomed moustache is now optional.

They are the ones responsible for the running of the entire hospital within an allocated budget. They have a system for this which works out that a stay in hospital should preferably cost no more than a jar of instant coffee per week. This works fine if every unfortunate brings his or her own camp bed, linen, food and medicines. They provide everything else.

This gift for merchandising medical care should come as no surprise when you learn that two years earlier they were trainee accountants or cracking the managerial whip in Woolworths. Asking irritating questions beginning with "Why is this patient..." will get you nowhere until you use the magic word 'unit' instead. Talk in terms of "cost per unit" and "unit turnover" and you will capture their full attention.

The friendly face of management can sometimes be seen engaging in heart-warming stunts like swapping jobs (not wages) with a cleaner for the day. They like to be seen everywhere, mucking in, so if you see someone fainting and clutching a clipboard in the operating theatre, don't worry, it's a manager. It's not the blood that gets them, it's the expense.

DUTIES

Your main duties as a junior hospital doctor will take you to:

The Wards

In large hospitals, you can easily find your way around the maze of wards by their numbers. Older hospitals, however, often have wards named after their distinguished benefactors or names that the founders thought appropriate at the time such as 'Gerontius Ward' for geriatric medicine or 'van Gogh Memorial Ward' for ear surgery.

In the future, the health service may wish to solve its financial problems by having ward sponsorship by interested parties. Doctors could easily find themselves working on the 'Nintendo Paediatric Unit' or, the 'Yamaha 650 Male Trauma Unit' and the 'Cosy Slippers Unit for the Elderly'.

When you arrive there, for your convenience you will find all the patients in the wards in rows like geraniums, neatly displayed and labelled. This is for your information as well as patient security. Anyone found wandering the corridors in their pyjamas can be identified and swiftly returned to their proper abode, just by reading their wristband: 'Name: Hague. Lost marbles. Ward 14.'

The arrangement of beds in long rows, like a Victorian workhouse, is called a 'Nightingale Ward', partly in deference to the famous Florence but mainly because nothing much has been changed since the Crimean War. In this hive of healing, you will do most of your work and find most of your customers. As new patients arrive there, it is the house officer's job to 'admit' them. This is called 'clerking' and consists of the initial interview and physical examination of the patient. The process may be repeated many times, day and night, and becomes an almost automatic process of information gleaning. This goes some way to explaining why, when you meet some doctors socially, they say 'Hello, and what's wrong with you then?' even before you shake hands.

At least once a week all the patients are visited by consultants and their entourage in the notorious **Ward Round**. This is a formal procession with the consultant leading like a mother duck and the lowly house officer bringing up the rear. In some teaching establishments this parade is deified as 'The Grand Round'. All that is missing is some suitably stirring music like the 'Pomp and Circumstance' march to make the occasion complete.

Patients and staff are on their best behaviour. This traditional healing ceremony is performed with military precision and with only slightly less reverence than a pilgrimage to Lourdes. Every patient gets to meet their consultant and some even get to touch the hem of their garment.

Consequently, in preparation, startled patients will have bedpans prematurely removed, their hair neatly combed and their Sunday dentures in and gleaming. Patients in possession of interesting signs and symptoms would do well to hide in the WCs until it's all over, unless they enjoy being the centre of attention. Once the ward round has passed, the patients breathe a sigh of relief and get on with the business of getting better.

As the house officer this is your opportunity to shine and you will be congratulated if all goes uneventfully. So, even if the rest of the week has been complete chaos, it pays triple-score points if you prepare for this spectacle so as to avoid any last minute surprises. When it comes to mistakes, unlike most seniority ladders, the buck stops well and truly with you.

Outpatients

This is where patients visit the hospital to attend a specialist clinic. People attending these clinics always complain to you that they never see the same doctor twice. Tell them that their malady is so interesting that there is a queue of different doctors waiting to see them every week.

Casualty

The doctor in casualty is expected to examine, diagnose and treat more patients per hour than the average person serving in McDonald's. Most of the time is taken up with the 'walking wounded', aches and pains, cuts and bruises and peanuts in children's ears. The nightmare sequelae of major accidents happen occasionally, but with prior warning the forward-thinking doctor will have enough assistance and expertise around to cope with the casualties of trench warfare.

Casualty doctors work in shifts and Saturday night is known as 'Pit Duty'. It's the night for every high-spirited youth to get dolled up, eat their own weight in curry, wash it down with about 20 pints of lager and pick a fight with a policeman. Multiply this by 20 and the waiting room soon looks like the aftermath of the Charge of the Light Brigade.

The good news is that if there is any stitching to be done on these inebriates they don't have to have any anaesthetic. They have already got enough on board for you to perform major surgery.

Weekends in casualty are also the time when people turn up with very minor complaints or something that they have had for months but 'didn't want to bother' their busy doctor with on his day off.

The layout of a casualty department into small cubicles known as 'traps' offers little in the way of privacy, and patients can often be heard broadcasting their intimate ailments to all and sundry from behind the curtains. The most common complaint you will have to deal with as the duty casualty doctor is 'Why have I had to wait so bloody long?'

At the end of eight hours of this you feel like walking into moving traffic. The only thing that stops you is the depressing thought that the ambulance would just bring you straight back in again.

Maternity

For some reason this area of the hospital strikes terror into the hearts of all but the most experienced doctors. It is the domain of the midwife, a 'specialist in her own right', and the doctor's role here is vital – to keep out of the way and to make the tea.

If a birth is difficult you don't have long to swing into action. When all is bearing down upon you, your role is to radiate serenity while phoning the duty consultant. If he is not at home then his wife might have an idea of what to do for the best; failing that you could try asking the patient's mother or the woman in the next room or one of the cleaners.

Keep calm at all times and try not to be intimidated by the fact that most experienced mothers have forgotten more than you'll ever learn about childbirth. Relax, and remember to breathe deeply but regularly.

Intensive (Expensive) Care Unit (ITU)

For the uninitiated this is like walking into NASA by mistake. Somewhere under a mass of plastic tubing and electronic gadgetry is the patient in your care.

Unless it's absolutely unavoidable, try not to take your hands out of your pockets, and above all resist the urge to twiddle with any knobs. Being the only one in your home who can set the video is no qualification for impulsively retuning some poor soul's vital functions. You may wish to justify your presence, however, by commenting on at least one piece of bedside apparatus: "I see this radio receives both Long wave and FM frequencies".

There is an unofficial maxim called the 'Rule of Five'. If more than five orifices have been obscured by plastic devices the situation may be regarded as 'critical'. If the patient is being ventilated by machine, look at the dials and say knowledgeably 'The tidal volume (size of each breath) looks adequate'; then look at the Electrocardiogram (the screen with the wiggly lines) to see if the heart is maintaining normal rate and rhythm. If it's banging out a rhythm like a samba you might want to get hold of someone who knows what they're doing.

If the patient is receiving fluids artificially through a vein, look at the catheter bag draining the patient's urine and hold it up to the light admiringly like a wine connoisseur. That's the quality taken care of, now for the quantity. Roughly speaking, if what is being poured in doesn't equal the amount coming out then your patient is retaining fluid and kidney failure is a possible diagnosis.

Be prepared for even your most rudimentary medical knowledge to desert you as you cross this hi-tech threshold and after five minutes you may even be mistaken for a concerned relative. If this happens, ask the sister if you can freshen the flowers or something and slip out.

Operating Theatre

Those engaged in performing the operation are 'scrubbed'. That is, they are covered in green gowns, surgical gloves and masks to avoid infecting the patient. The rest of the theatre staff not directly involved with the operation are 'unscrubbed' and thus 'dirty' as far as surgery is concerned. The dirtiest of these is invariably the anaesthetist who has to think of something stimulating to keep himself awake.

As a junior you will be required to assist the

surgeon in such exciting tasks as cutting sutures to the required length and holding bits of surgical ironmongery for hours, well away from the interesting bits. When your mind is sufficiently far removed, the surgeon will usually ask you to identify a portion of anatomy that looks as if a hyena has been at it.

Try to recall those far-off days of dissecting dead bodies. If you don't know, take a wild guess but try not to say 'ovaries' or 'uterus' if the patient has a chin full of stubble.

Post Mortem Room

Most junior doctors eventually find themselves here to discover what went wrong with their less than successful cases. Here the pathologist takes a leisurely stroll through the innards of the deceased and gives the definitive diagnosis.

If you weren't even close and your ego can't take it then this is when the doctor's unreadable handwriting ploy comes into its own and, pointing to your scribbled notes, you can show that you were right all along. Your colleagues will be impressed with the unswerving accuracy of your diagnostic powers and the patient will be past the stage of giving evidence to the contrary.

SKILLS TO MASTER

Patient Spotting

As the first doctor that the patients see on coming to hospital, you must quickly learn the art of **Triage**. This is basically sorting those who are seriously ill from those who are a bit off colour, and all shades in between.

The seasoned veteran has learned that some patients part only reluctantly with the clues to their diagnosis. The patient with the severe central chest pain of a heart attack may confess to "a slight twinge after eating pickled onions". Those who minimise their symptoms, often so as "not to bother you", are more than compensated for by those who give an Oscar-winning deathbed performance with an ingrowing toenail.

Only time will reveal to you the meaning of 'patient-speak'. Anything from a touch of shingles to raging paranoid schizophrenia will be covered by 'trouble with the nerves'. Similarly, 'one of those funny spells' naturally embraces anything from a full blown stroke to a victim of witchcraft. Watch out for those trying to be helpful with the medications they take: "The tablets used to be blue but now they're pink and they fizz."

If someone gives it to you on a plate with "I've got a cardiac heart, doctor", look out for the rest of the anatomical syndromes, renal kidneys, cerebral brain and a gastric stomach.

By way of revenge, doctors don't always tell the truth either. Many a patient has had to be held down though the last thing the doctor said was "This won't hurt a bit".

Children are not so gullible. No matter what you

say, they treat you with the suspicion normally afforded to a time-share salesman.

Impromptu Doctoring

Whether in a theatre, a supermarket or 'al fresco' by the side of the road, the cry 'Is there a doctor here?' should strike joy into the heart of any member of the medical profession. Here is the much dreamed of chance to apply those hard learned skills, and shine.

Move into action confidently and if there isn't a phone box nearby where you can quickly change into your white coat, don't panic. Walk purposely forward saying the magic words "Let me through, I'm a doctor". With a bit of luck, by the time you've got your jacket off and ferreted around in your bag for your stethoscope, the patient will have recovered enough to thank you for saving his life. But if you are hopelessly heroic in temperament, make sure you have individual malpractice insurance which will cover you should that elderly rich widow from Florida decide that since you felt her pulse on the plane, she can no longer drive her Cadillac.

Cardiac Arrest

This is an urgent summons to someone in the hospital whose heart has inadvertently stopped. With your bleep sounding like an air-raid siren, join the rest of the cavalry charge down the corridors to give aid.

As a general rule, all such emergencies take place in the opposite end of the hospital from where you happen to be. When you arrive, panting for breath, it is considered bad form to snatch the oxygen from the patient to revive yourself first. The general idea is to assemble as much medical expertise in under three minutes around the inactive organ and 'bump start' it again. Sometimes the shock of seeing ten doctors arriving all at once is enough to do the trick.

Bedside Manners

This may be broadly defined as the way in which the attending physician behaves just being around the patient. This 'presence' which surrounds the experienced doctor is supposed to raise the patient's morale and the chances of getting better long before anything medical has been done. Whether the patient rises like Lazarus or slips slowly and inevitably towards a meeting with St Peter, the wise will remember that often it is not what they do or say but how they are seen to perform that matters.

A 'poor bedside manner' usually involves one or more of these cardinal breaches of etiquette:

1. Failing to introduce yourself before you start asking intimate questions and examining the patient. The white coat is not self explanatory – you could be painting the corridor.

2. Interrogating patients like a KGB officer because they aren't giving the right answers to your questions.

3. Looking bored when you've heard it all before. It's the only story they've got.

4. Whipping back the covers to examine someone's cheeky bits without asking permission. Never mix

social and professional behaviour.

5. Being too technical. "This rash you had, was it macular or papular?" You are the one with the medical degree.

6. Being too colloquial when explaining things, like "We're just going to put this clever telescope up your bottom." The last telescope they saw was probably about two feet long with an end on it the size of a marrow.

7. Being condescending with children. Common offenders are aspiring anaesthetists. The last thing kids want to hear as they go off to sleep is: "I'm just going to pass wind in front of your face."

Like a true apprenticeship the art of good doctoring will be learned only after many years and many such diplomatic gaffs.

Tools of the Trade

Handwriting

It is now traditional that whenever a doctor puts pen to paper, the resultant scrawl should keep a graphologist (or an infant teacher) happy for about a week. As a rule, the more important the contents, the more enigmatic the scribbling should be.

Once the words have been deciphered, there is the schoolboy Latin to unboggle. After all, if mere mortals knew that 'Unct. Top. tds.' meant spread the ointment on three times a day, it would lose all its magic.

Stethoscope

Don't underestimate the significance of this few feet of rubber tubing. It is your 'chain of office', so wear it with pride. In some doctors' hands (or ears) that is about as useful as it gets. If the vibrations of the patient's breathing or the sounds of the heart are just meaningless noise to you, don't fret. When the ear-pieces are in position you can have two minutes of uninterrupted silence while you think of something suitable to say.

Ophthalmoscope

This glorified torch allows you to inspect the inside of the patient's eyes and, in the hands of the experienced, diseases such as diabetes and high blood pressure may be detected. Even if you are not this good with it, because you have to lean so close to the patient's face, you can at least diagnose a case of roaring halitosis.

Auriscope

Another torch – this time for looking in the ears. With most patients, the most exciting thing you will see is wax which looks rather like an extreme close up of the contents of a jar of Marmite.

Rubber Gloves

Just the sound of the doctor snapping gloves on is enough to strike fear into the bowels of any patient. If they are giving you a hard time, put them on and you will get their undivided attention.

FLIES IN THE OINTMENT

The Bleep

This electronic albatross is the bane of every doctor's life. When you first get one it is a visible, and audible, sign of your importance and indispensability. After about two days you want to lose it – permanently.

It is possible however, to set it off yourself, with a deft flick of a switch, if you find yourself trapped in an awkward situation for too long.

On the other hand the more paranoid know that personal pagers are programmed to bleep when brought into proximity with food, congenial company of the opposite sex or soft furnishings, especially beds, and that if placed near all three at once they go off like a burglar alarm.

The Hours

The law limits the number of hours worked by a bus or train driver for safety reasons and doctors are not supposed to work in excess of 72 hours a week. However, many junior doctors still find themselves working anything from 60–100 hours a week. Being unable to think rationally because of lack of sleep isn't thought to be a problem.

Britain is the only advanced country that still uses this archaic 'Doc till you Drop' system. Having to work this many hours is supposed to be so that doctors in training can experience a wide range of medical conditions during the course of their early years. As a fully paid up member of the walking dead, the only conditions that they end up knowing really well are sleep-walking and exhaustion.

The Pay

Anyone who whinges about doctors being underpaid will be criticised for being unprofessional. You are paid in something called 'job satisfaction' which doesn't involve money. Don't ask why you can't have both.

This fits in nicely with working long hours because you never have time to spend anything. It is advisable to have someone handy with the smelling salts when you get your first pay cheque. Look at the box for unsocial hours' pay and you will see more Zeros than there were at Pearl Harbour.

IT (Information Technology)

Doctors are now expected to understand and use IT. This means needing computer skills to read your patient's medical records or order a set of blood tests for them. There have already been link-up consultations between hospital based specialists and GPs' surgeries via computerised web cameras. Visualise lots of patients exposing their uvulas and saying "Ahhhh" or showing their back passages to the camera in the interests of science. Worse, your patients will have access to information about their ailments from the Internet and will be demanding the same marvellous treatment that Mrs Kleinberg had for her varicose veins in Seattle last week.

The Accommodation

All junior doctors are expected to live in the hospital residency for at least the first year. It is colloquially known, as in the army, as the 'Mess'. This name did not arise by accident. It comprises a collection of doctors' bedrooms with some optional extras such as bathrooms and laundry rooms, and essentials such as the snooker room and bar.

Bedrooms are very basic and all the furniture is G-plan, as in Gulag. Don't worry about the fact that the bed is narrow and lumpy because you won't be doing much sleeping on it. The designers have thought of that and made the walls so thin you can hear your neighbour flossing his teeth.

Add to this an orchestra of activated bleeps, round the clock loud music and door-banging, and you get the picture. On the whole, mess life is a blend of living with The Waltons and being locked up in Cell Block H.

Big Brother

Traditionalists may be outraged, but the general public and the government want more of a say in how you practice medicine. The tired old NHS, born in 1948, is being overhauled to make it 'leaner and fitter' and the tablets coming down the mountain from the Department of Health have catchy titles like 'Putting Patients First' and 'Fit for the Future'.

Ideas include **Clinical Governance**, a wide ranging system of quality controls, and **standards** set for everything from waiting times for appointments to the speed taken to respond to granny's needs with a commode. The **Patients' Charter** sets out your customers' rights and a motley gang of bruisers called **patients' advocates** will argue for them. Your competence, level of current knowledge, and ability to deliver the modes of treatment enshrined in the manuals of **Evidence Based Practice** will be monitored with yearly **CPD** (Continual Professional Develop-ment) assessments. Duffers who have only just got the hang of this new fangled penicillin thing will be out quicker than a badly inserted suppository.

The Social Life

The mess bar is the focal point of any residency. These medical watering holes often have names like 'The Foot Drop Inn' or 'The Call of Nature'. Here you will find a motley collection of off-duty junior doctors and some seniors who should know better.

Attendance at the formal 'Mess Dinners' is mandatory. They take place only on 'special' occasions such as Christmas, Spring, Burns Night, Anzac Day, the Queen's Birthday, the D-Day landings, Norwegian Independence Day, any Mess member's birthday, and just about any other day that seems appropriate. It is a formal bacchanalia but you can expect to see the normally serious and stuffy consultant mutate into an expert in limbo dancing or down a Yard of Ale in record time while standing on his head.

Romance

This is the stuff that makes hearts beat faster and a fortune for Mills & Boon. The basic plot rarely varies. A rich, brilliant doctor fresh from medical school forsakes his family fortune and devotes his life to healing the sick. He meets a student nurse over a warm bedpan and she changes his whole life. After he has found a cure (any cure) he decides to take his money and use it to get married and open a medical mission in Africa.

If junior doctors could get out of the hospital once in a while to meet the rest of the human race none of this 'doctor meets nurse' would have to happen. In truth, male doctors marry the only women that they come into contact with, nurses and barmaids.

ALTERNATIVE MEDICINE

There is nothing like a training in Western conventional medicine to induce a more than healthy scepticism about any alternative way of going about things. You didn't spend five gruelling years in the hallowed places of medical learning to emerge with your new qualification and admit magnanimously that you only got part of the story. However, when the dust has gathered on your diploma a little and you're working in the middle of the night yet again, any alternative whatsoever seems appealing.

The fees for such alternative practitioners are lucrative. You can train in Homeopathy, Acupuncture or Reflexology which take time, applied skill and practice. A period studying Aromatherapy would seem like a breath of fresh air after five years on the hospital wards inhaling nothing but Dettol and discarded bowel gas. The arduous requirements for a diploma in Crystal-therapy are a large cheque and a stamped addressed envelope.

The Media Doctor

Through the miracle of newspapers, magazines, national television and bad taste, you can now conduct a long-distance surgery with millions of people. In trendy magazines with such appropriate titles as *Women's Monthly* you can advise in your column about the hazards of hormone therapy, bedwetting and flat feet, or put someone's mind at rest when they find their husband dressed up like a French maid. Why these people never go and ask their own doctor's advice but prefer to wait three weeks for a reply to come through the post is none of your business.

You may even get an emergency enquiry such as "I have just severed an artery on a sharp object and I am rapidly losing consciousness. Please advise." Your training should immediately tell you that the reply should be posted with a first-class stamp.

More photogenic doctors may get a chance to hold a phone-in surgery on breakfast television. Looking professionally at the camera you can thank a viewer for her urine sample of last week and congratulate her on her pregnancy; and if someone asks you a hard one and you can't think of a reply on the spot, the professional teledoctor will smile and say, "Take two aspirins and watch again tomorrow."

GLOSSARY

Alternative medicine – What you try when all else fails.

Appendicectomy – The removal of the appendix. Often the first operation performed by newly qualified doctors. Normally a very quick procedure, theatre staff have been known to change shifts

Admission – A new patient entering the hospital (common) or a doctor giving a straight answer to a question (rare).

Anaemic – Pale and interesting.

Ash-cash – The fee paid to a doctor for completing a cremation form.

Bloods – The series of laboratory investigations carried out when a patient first enters hospital.

Chapel – The hospital doctor's bar where many a chalice is raised at vespers after work.

Clerk – Old term for a house physician.

Dresser – Old term for a house surgeon.

Drug store – The hospital pharmacy.

'-ectomy' – Anything with this on the end of it will be removed, surgically speaking.

Elective – A non-urgent procedure that has been booked into hospital; or the period a student spends, usually abroad, during training.

Emergency – A medical situation that won't wait till you've finished your chips/beer.

Foot and Mouth – The back end of the hospital where the Chiropody and Dental Departments are located.

Gonner – Someone who has undergone a **TME** (q.v.).

Heartbreak hotel – The Coronary Care Unit

Iatrogenic – A condition arising from medical treatment (from the Greek; Iatros = Physician).

Laparotomy – Stem to stern abdominal operation done when you're not sure what the problem is. A general 'kit inspection', with a scar to match.

NHS – National Health Service introduced in 1948, now thought to stand for No Hope of Survival.

Milk of amnesia – Brew served in the doctor's mess.

Munchausen's syndrome – A psychiatric disorder where the sufferer constantly pretends to be ill.

Medical phobia – An understandable disorder when the sufferer constantly pretends to be well.

Murmur – The sound of a broken heart through a stethoscope.

Oligoneuronal – A cerebrally challenged person.

On call – Period the doctor works out of office hours.

The Operation – When spoken in a whisper by elderly ladies, a hysterectomy.

Placebo – Physiologically inactive medication that works because the doctor says so.

Plants/pictures – Temporary hospital furniture which appears from nowhere when there is an important visitor.

Plumbus oscillans (swinging the lead) – Diagnosis

made when a patient is being economical with the truth.

Privates – Paying patients, or genitals.

Premature ejaculation – Speaking too soon.

Primum non nocere ('First of all, do no harm') – The L-plates of all newly qualified doctors.

Regular – A state of intestinal 'nirvana' where the patient's bowels are synchronised with the rotation of the earth.

Syndrome – A specific collection of symptoms and signs of a disease.

Supratentorially deficient – Another term for someone with a brain like a 15 watt bulb.

TME – A Terminal Morbid Event (death) in medical statisticians' language, or what American doctors would refer to as a 'negative ongoing life experience'.

THC (Three Hots and a Cot) – Minimal care (i.e. three hot meals and a bed) for someone in hospital.

Triage – The sorting of cases in order of importance.

UMTs (Units of Medical Time) – What is used to calculate doctors' salaries. Should more accurately be called Underpaid Mandatory Time.

Viva – A spoken examination.

Ward round – The weekly tour (it only seems to last for two days) made by consultants to all patients in their care.

Whip round – The charitable gleaning of money by good souls for hospital luxuries such as kidney machines, operating equipment and beds.

THE AUTHOR

Patrick Keating was born in Dublin in 1953 and can remember nothing prior to that date.

He attended school in Yorkshire and was the finest centre half and boy soprano that Whitby Road Junior ever produced, but had eventually to give up both activities due to sudden loss of ball control.

His future in the medical profession seemed assured from the age of ten when his essay 'Things I want to do when I grow up' forced his teacher Miss Machin to take early retirement.

He acquired his degree in Medicine in 1980 through the post while working as a pool attendant in Forth Worth, Texas, and he has pursued his career with the same dogged enthusiasm ever since.

He is currently engaged in medical research into the marked correlation between pre-senile dementia and voting Conservative.